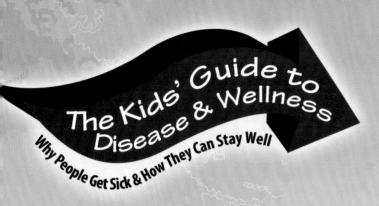

The Kids' Guide to Disease & Wellness
Why People Get Sick & How They Can Stay Well

POLLUTION CAN MAKE YOU SICK!

The Kids' Guide to Disease & Wellness:
Why People Get Sick and How They Can Stay Well
POLLUTION CAN MAKE YOU SICK!

Copyright © 2009 by AlphaHouse Publishing, a division of PEMG Publishing Group.
All rights reserved. No part of this publication may be reproduced or transmitted
in any form or by any means, electronic or mechanical, including photocopying,
recording, taping, or any information storage and retrieval system, without
permission from the publisher.

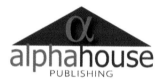

AlphaHouse Publishing
201 Harding Avenue
Vestal, NY 13850

First Printing

9 8 7 6 5 4 3 2 1

ISBN: 978-1-934970-13-3
ISBN (series): 978-1-934970-11-9
   Library of Congress Control Number:
   2008930670

Author: Simons, Rae

Cover design by MK Bassett-Harvey.
Interior and cover design by MK Bassett-Harvey
and Wendy Baker.

Printed in India by International Print-O-Pac Limited

 An ISO 9001 Company

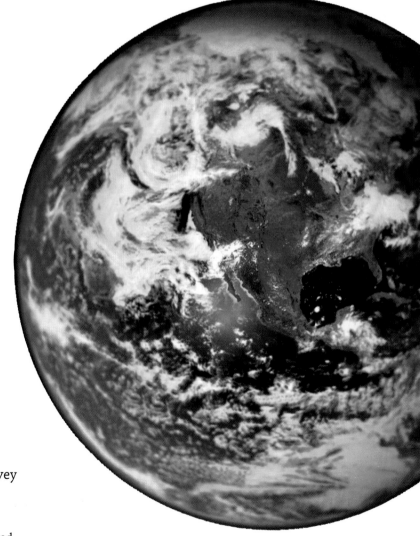

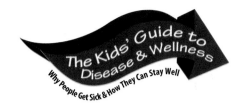

The Kids' Guide to
Disease & Wellness

Why People Get Sick & How They Can Stay Well

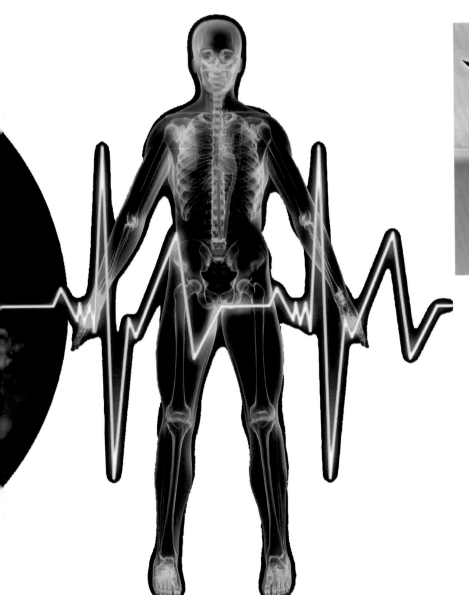

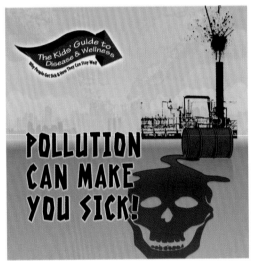

POLLUTION
CAN MAKE
YOU SICK!

By Rae Simons

SERIES LIST

Bugs Can Make You Sick!

Pollution Can Make You Sick!

Cancer & Kids

Why Can't I Breathe? Kids & Asthma

Things You Can't See Can Make You Sick: Viruses and Bacteria

Kids & Diabetes

What Causes Allergies?

Malnutrition & Kids

AIDS & HIV: The Facts for Kids

Immunizations: Saving Lives

INTRODUCTION

According to a recent study reported in the Virginia Henderson International Nursing Library, kids worry about getting sick. They worry about AIDS and cancer, about allergies and the "super-germs" that resist medication. They know about these ills—but they don't always understand what causes them or how they can be prevented.

Unfortunately, most 9- to 11–year–olds, the study found, get their information about diseases like AIDS from friends and television; only 20 percent of the children interviewed based their understanding of illness on facts they had learned at school. Too often, kids believe urban legends, schoolyard folktales, and exaggerated movie plots. Oftentimes, misinformation like this only makes their worries worse. The January 2008 *Child Health News* reported that 55 percent of all children between 9 and 13 "worry almost all the time" about illness.

This series, **The Kids' Guide to Disease and Wellness**, offers readers clear information on various illnesses and conditions, as well as the immunizations that can prevent many diseases. The books dispel the myths with clearly presented facts and colorful, accurate illustrations. Better yet, these books will help kids understand not only illness—but also what they can do to stay as healthy as possible.

—*Dr. Elise Berlan*

JUST THE FACTS

- There are three main kinds of pollution: air pollution, water pollution, and land pollution.

- Pollution can make people sick because they are connected with the Earth and the environment.

- Pollution in the air, like particles from burning coal or wood, can harm your lungs, eyes, and throat.

- Air pollution can cause asthma, heart disease, and even cancer.

- Pollution in water can be dangerous when people drink water that is unclean or contains chemicals.

- Water pollution can cause disease, especially when industrial waste is dropped into the water people drink.

- Soil can become polluted when people bury waste, use chemical pesticides, or dump garbage into landfills.

- Global warming has many negative effects on the environment and human health, including increases in disease, air pollution, and extreme weather.

- It is important to consider ways you can help preserve the environment, including recycling, using cars less, and being aware of the electricity you're using.

WHAT IS POLLUTION?

Pollution is what happens when we make our world dirty. Sometimes it's easy to see the dirt we've put into our environment—like when the sky over a city looks yellow and cloudy, or when water is green and smells bad. But other times, pollution is invisible. We may not be able to see the chemicals in the air, water, or land, but they are there, and they can kill the Earth's plants and wildlife.

The three main kinds of pollution are:

• air pollution
• water pollution
• land pollution

Global warming is another problem that's also caused by pollution.

Although sometimes nature causes pollution—like when a flood washes dirt into a lake—the Earth can usually handle the pollution caused by natural events such as storms and floods. Most times, though, people cause pollution. Factories like the ones in this picture put chemicals and tiny particles of dirt into the air and water. Cars, trucks, and airplanes produce air pollution. Even our farms often put dangerous

WORDS TO KNOW

Ecosystem: All the living and nonliving things in a particular area, including rocks, soil, plants, and animals.

8

chemicals into the land and water. And then there's our garbage! So many human activities—from eating a candy bar to wrapping a birthday gift—produce waste that has to be put somewhere. All this garbage usually ends up in landfills.

Pollution isn't bad just for the Earth, though. It's bad for people, too.

DID YOU KNOW?

Another kind of pollution is noise pollution. Too much noise can also hurt our environment. Noise can upset the balance of natural ecosystems. This kind of pollution can hurt human health, too, because it can damage our hearing. Being around loud noises—like the sound of machinery or jets—can also add stress to people's lives. Doctors have even found that high noise levels can raise people's blood pressure, creating a health risk.

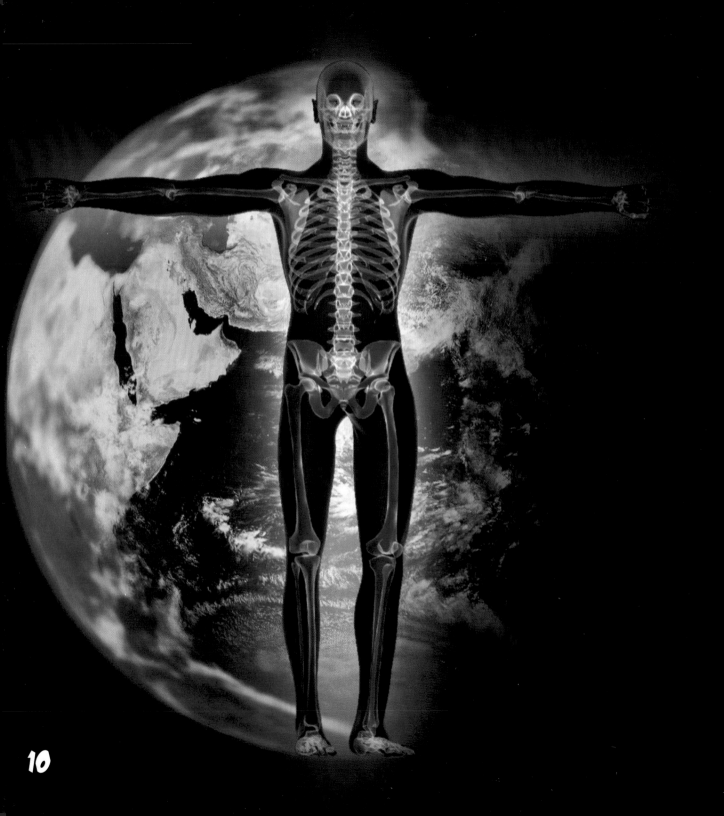

WHY DOES POLLUTION MAKE PEOPLE SICK?

Pollution makes people sick because all that dirt and garbage OUTSIDE ends up INSIDE our bodies.

Once upon a time, people thought of the Earth as though it were their mother. They loved Mother Earth and they respected her. They tried to understand her better. They knew that human beings need the Earth for food and water and air. They understood that if the Earth is sick, humans will be sick, too—and if the Earth dies, so will we!

Nowadays, many of us think that food comes from the store, already packaged in plastic or cardboard. We forget that everything we eat came from the land, from plants and animals. We think of water as something that comes out of the faucet whenever we want it—and we forget that it comes from lakes and streams, from rainfall and snowfall, and from the sea. We inhale in the air around us, and we don't think about what we're putting into our lungs.

Pollution makes us sick because we can't separate our lives from the Earth's. Everything we eat, drink, breathe, and touch once came from the Earth. Because the outside world ends up inside our bodies, we need to keep Mother Earth healthy!

WORDS TO KNOW

Inhale: to breathe in.

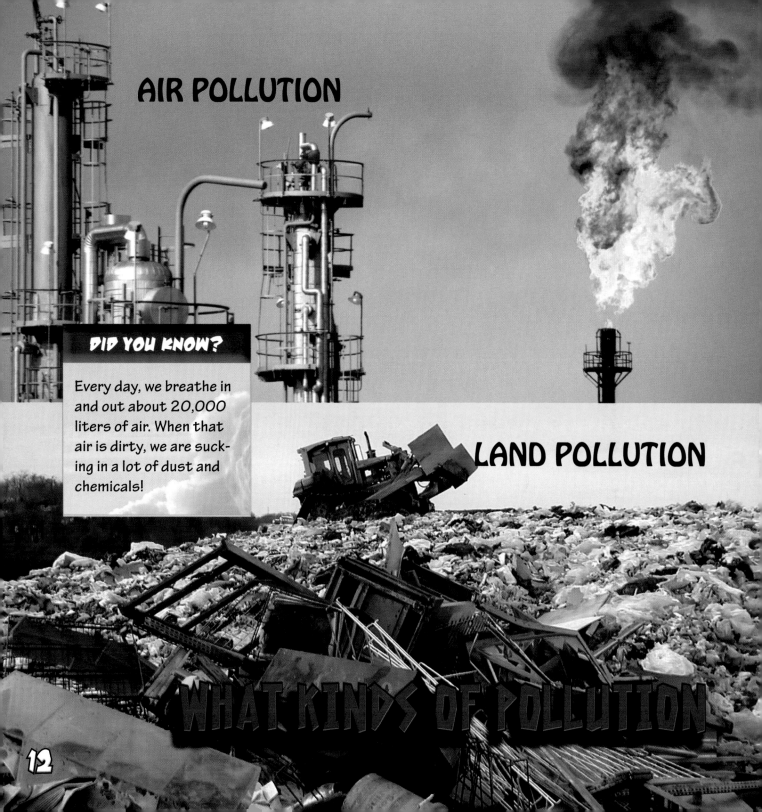

AIR POLLUTION

DID YOU KNOW?

Every day, we breathe in and out about 20,000 liters of air. When that air is dirty, we are sucking in a lot of dust and chemicals!

LAND POLLUTION

WHAT KINDS OF POLLUTION

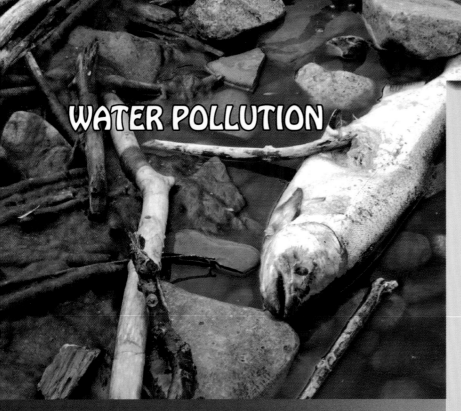

WATER POLLUTION

WORDS TO KNOW

Global warming: the gradual increase of the Earth's average air, land, and water temperatures, caused by humans putting pollution into the air. The dirty air acts like a greenhouse, holding in the Earth's heat so that it cannot escape as quickly into space.

GLOBAL WARMING

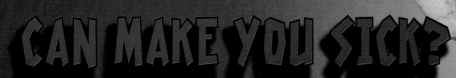

CAN MAKE YOU SICK?

AIR POLLUTION AND YOUR BODY

My family and I got stuck in a traffic jam inside a tunnel. The air smelled really bad and it gave me a headache. Am I going to get sick from breathing all that car exhaust?

A: Although constantly breathing polluted air can make you sick, most healthy people who are exposed for a short time to pollution like this will feel better as soon as the air improves. If you notice any problems with your breathing, though, let an adult know. If the problem doesn't go away soon, you may need to see your doctor.

Air pollution can make your eyes, throat, and lungs sore. Your chest may feel tight or you may cough. Because exercise requires faster, deeper breathing, it may make these symptoms worse. Some people are more sensitive to pollution than others.

Air pollution can make you sick in different ways. And it's not just outdoor air that can harm you—indoor air can also be polluted.

WHAT HAPPENS INSIDE YOUR BODY WHEN THERE'S POLLUTION OUTSIDE YOUR BODY?

Tiny particles from burning gasoline, coal, and wood can go deep into a person's lungs and from there get into the bloodstream. When they do, they increase the chance of heart attack, lung cancer, and stroke. Air pollution can irritate the lungs and make a person more likely to get some form of lung disease, such as pneumonia, asthma, or cancer.

WORDS TO KNOW

Stroke: bleeding in the brain, which can cause serious health problems, including death.

Pneumonia: an infection where fluid collects in the lungs.

15

ASTHMA

For most people, breathing is simple. They breathe air in through their noses or mouths, and the air goes into the windpipe, down through the windpipe (the trachea) into the bronchial tubes, and from there into the lungs—and then back out again. But for people with asthma, breathing can be a problem sometimes. During an asthma attack, the bronchial tubes can become swollen. Sometimes the lungs fill up with sticky mucus. When this happens, taking in a breath and letting it out can become very hard. Sometimes, it's almost impossible. People with asthma need to take special medicine to keep this from happening—and when it does happen, they need another kind of medicine to help their breathing go back to normal. Not being able to breathe can feel pretty scary.

An asthma attack is usually caused by a "trigger." It could be a change in air temperature or it could be an emotion, like when you get really angry. A lot of the time, though, triggers are substances in the air, like pollen from plants, hair from a pet—or pollution. The

WORDS TO KNOW

Bronchial tubes: the air passageways that lead from your windpipe into your lungs.

Mucus: a thick, slippery fluid that iines certain parts of the body, including the nose and throat.

Ozone: a gas produced when sunlight combines with chemicals made by cars and factories.

DID YOU KNOW?

Around the world, about 150 million people have asthma. It is most common in North America and Europe—and least common in rural Africa. This makes scientists suspect that people are more apt to get asthma when they breathe in pollution from cars and factories.

two kinds of air pollution that are most apt to trigger an asthma attack are ozone (found in smog) and particle pollution (found in smoke and dust).

Asthma used to be rare, but now it is becoming more common than it ever was before. Doctors suspect that this is because of air pollution. Not only does air pollution trigger asthma attacks, but it makes you more likely to develop asthma in the first place.

Children are especially likely to get asthma. In North America, asthma is now one of the most common illnesses in children; 1 child in every 15 has it. This means that if you were in a class with 15 students, at least one of you would probably have asthma. Why do so many children get asthma? It may be partly because they are more likely than adults to be outside, running around.

People who have asthma will always have asthma. It's not a disease you outgrow—but that doesn't mean if you have asthma that you will always have symptoms. Asthma medicines help keep the bronchial tubes from becoming narrow. Learning what triggers asthma attacks and avoiding those situations can also help a person with asthma control the symptoms.

One of the best ways to prevent asthma, though, may be to clean up our air!

ASK THE DOCTOR

If I have asthma, does that mean I can't play sports?
A: No, it doesn't mean that at all. In fact, exercise can actually improve your lung function—and many athletes have asthma. But because you have asthma, you need to be sure you take whatever medicines your doctor has prescribed, especially while exercising. (Make sure you tell your doctor you want to play sports.) And when the air quality is bad (for instance, on a hot day when the air is unusually smoggy), you may want to stay indoors or at least avoid exercising until smog levels go down. This is because exercise requires that you suck more air into your lungs—and you don't want more ozone in there!

HEART DISEASE

Scientist have found that the very small particles in dust, soot, and smoke can damage your heart. When you breathe in these tiny pieces of dirt, they pass from your lungs into your blood, and from there they travel to other parts of your body, including your heart. Researchers have

WORDS TO KNOW

Heart disease: abnormal conditions that affect the heart, including hardening of the arteries within the heart; heart failure, when the heart cannot pump blood normally; and arrhythmias, changes in the rate of heartbeat.

found that this is especially dangerous when it's combined with a high-fat diet. People in North America are particularly at danger, because many of them breathe in lots of air pollution AND eat foods that are high in fat. The air pollution and the fatty diet combine to make blood vessels narrower and clogged. This condition can lead to heart disease.

Air pollution can be especially dangerous for people who already have heart disease. Doctors recommend that people with heart conditions avoid areas where air pollution is high. All of us should avoid exercising in areas where the air is more apt to be full of pollution. Instead or jogging or bicycling along busy streets, for example, go to a park. Find ways to exercise indoors when air pollution levels are especially high.

DID YOU KNOW?

Heart disease kills more than 7 million people each year. In North America, it is the leading cause of death for both men and women.

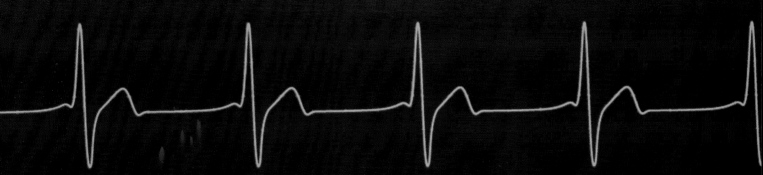

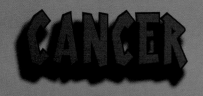

CANCER

Cancer is a disease where cells grow abnormally. When this happens, the cells may eventually form tumors, growths that can invade normal tissues and keep other organs from functioning the way they should.

Chemicals found in air pollution **OUTSIDE** can trigger the abnormal cell growth that causes cancer **INSIDE**. According to the U.S. Environmental Protection Agency, more than 175 million pounds of cancer-causing chemicals are released by factories into the air each year. (And scientists say that number is just the tip of the iceberg, because it doesn't include the air pollution from cars and trucks, airports, power plants, incinerators, and other smaller polluters.)

Children are especially affected by the chemicals found in air pollution. The toxic chemicals found in pollution can cause leukemia, as well as other kinds of childhood cancers.

It's not just the chemicals in air pollution that can

ASK THE DOCTOR

If I live in a city with lots of air pollution, am I doomed to get cancer?
A: No! Not everyone who is exposed to air pollution gets cancer. But your chances are greater than if you lived somewhere with cleaner air. However, there are things you can do to help protect your body against cancer, even if you have to breathe air pollution every day—and eating plenty of fruits and vegetables is one of the best things you can do. These foods contain vitamins and other compounds that help the body resist cancer.

Toxic: poisonous, harmful to life.

Leukemia: a kind of cancer where the body produces too many white blood cells.

cause cancer. The small particles found in pollution can also cause this deadly disease. This kind of pollution is especially apt to trigger lung cancer, which is the leading cause of deaths from cancer in North America. When you inhale smoke and other particle pollution, the tiny pieces of soot and dirt damage the lining of your lungs. At first, your body will repair this damage, but after enough time goes by, your body may not be able to keep up with the repair work. This is when cancer can develop inside the lungs. Eventually, the cancer can travel from the lungs to other parts of the body. Doctors say that a person who breathes polluted air for long periods of time is as much at risk of developing lung cancer as a person who lives with a cigarette smoker.

WATER POLLUTION AND YOU

Water pollution happens any time dirt or chemicals get into water, making it unfit for natural and human uses.

WORDS TO KNOW

Balance: when there is the right amount of all parts working together to keep something working the way it should.

WHAT DOES WATER POLLUTION LOOK LIKE ON THE **OUTSIDE**?

Water that is polluted may look brown or green, where clean water will be clear. You may see a film on top of the water. Sometimes you may not be able to see certain kinds of chemicals in water, but if water is clean, wildlife, including fish, salamanders, frogs, and many kinds of insects, will live there. Polluted water will be able to support only a few kinds of creatures (if any). With any ecosystem, it's important to keep the balance nature intended—and pollution can throw off this balance. For example, too many chemicals of a certain kind can make plants and algae grow too fast and thick in the water, which in turn puts chemicals in the water that are bad for fish and other animals.

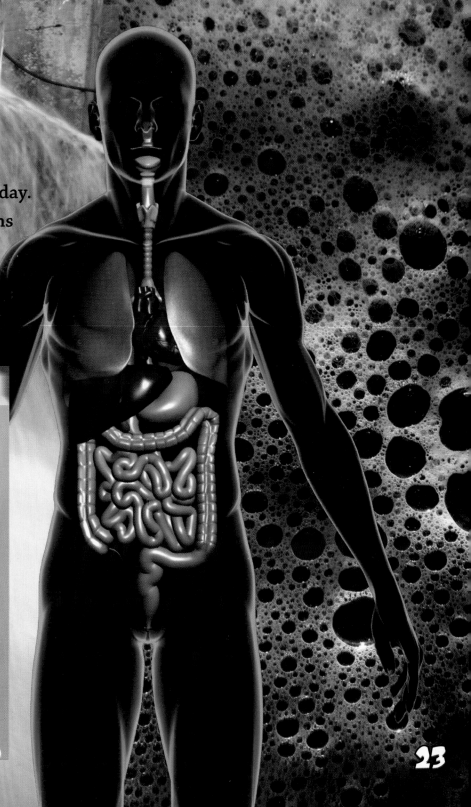

WHAT DOES WATER POLLUTION DO ON THE **INSIDE OF YOUR BODY?**

Your body needs water every day. If the water you drink contains pollution, germs and chemicals will enter your body. When they do, they can make you sick.

ASK THE DOCTOR

If my family drinks city water, it won't be polluted, right?

A: Probably not. Most cities in the United States, Canada, and much of Europe test their water carefully to make sure it is healthy. But the water you drink can also be polluted after it enters your house. Lead and copper from the pipes can get into drinking water and be very bad for you. Find out what kind of plumbing your house or apartment has. If the pipes are lead or copper, only use cold water for drinking and cooking, and let it run for a while before you use it.

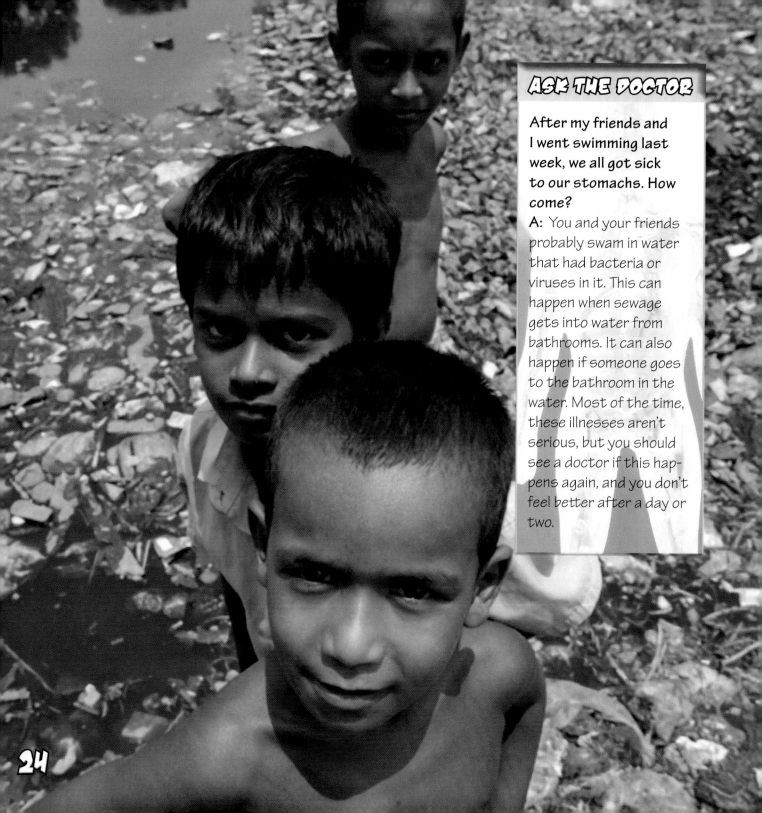

After my friends and I went swimming last week, we all got sick to our stomachs. How come?

A: You and your friends probably swam in water that had bacteria or viruses in it. This can happen when sewage gets into water from bathrooms. It can also happen if someone goes to the bathroom in the water. Most of the time, these illnesses aren't serious, but you should see a doctor if this happens again, and you don't feel better after a day or two.

WATER-BORNE DISEASES

Sometimes sewage from homes and farms leaks into the water supply. In some parts of the world, communities simply dump human and animal wastes into streams and lakes that are also used for bathing and drinking. When this happens, germs from the **OUTSIDE** can get **INSIDE** your body. Sometimes tiny one-celled animals like the ones shown in the picture to the right can live in water that's polluted, and these creatures can also make people sick.

Drinking or swimming in dirty water can give you a stomach ache and diarrhea, or make you throw up. Certain kinds of germs could also give you an itchy skin rash or a fever. Most of the time, these illnesses will make you feel uncomfortable, but you'll feel better soon. Other times, though, especially in parts of the world like Africa, Asia, and Latin America, polluted water can make you very, very sick. That's why it's a good idea to only drink bottled water when

WORDS TO KNOW

Sewage: the liquid and solid waste materials that animals and humans produce.

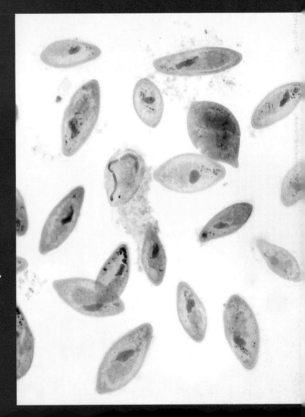

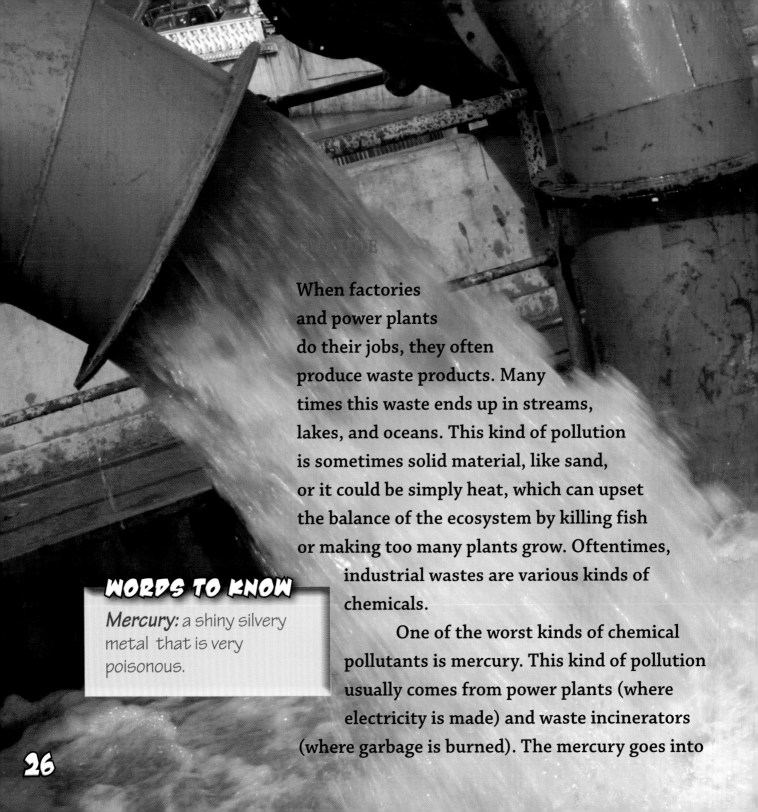

When factories
and power plants
do their jobs, they often
produce waste products. Many
times this waste ends up in streams,
lakes, and oceans. This kind of pollution
is sometimes solid material, like sand,
or it could be simply heat, which can upset
the balance of the ecosystem by killing fish
or making too many plants grow. Oftentimes,
industrial wastes are various kinds of
chemicals.

One of the worst kinds of chemical
pollutants is mercury. This kind of pollution
usually comes from power plants (where
electricity is made) and waste incinerators
(where garbage is burned). The mercury goes into

WORDS TO KNOW

Mercury: a shiny silvery metal that is very poisonous.

INDUSTRIAL WASTES

DID YOU KNOW?

The Industrial Revolution that took place in the 1700s is when mercury pollution began. Scientists believe that on average, there is three times more mercury being washed into the Earth's water today than there was before the Industrial Revolution.

the air, but then it falls to the ground. When it rains, the water washes over the ground and carries the mercury into streams and rivers. It gets inside fish— and it can get inside you if you eat that fish.

INSIDE

If even very small amounts of mercury get inside you, it can hurt your kidneys, liver, and brain. Your body cannot get rid of mercury by itself, which means it will gradually build up inside you. If it is not treated by a doctor, mercury poisoning causes pain, weakness, and loss of vision. Eventually, a person with mercury poisoning will not be able to move his muscles. He may even die.

Industries also dump other kinds of pollution into waterways. Sometimes, for example, petroleum gets in the water accidentally, like when a tanker ship carrying oil crashes and spills its load into the ocean. Other times, petroleum gets into the ocean from off-shore oil drilling. Oil spills like this are very dangerous to the wildlife that lives in and on the water. Even years later, sea creatures may still be affected by being exposed to petroleum pollution.

People can get sick when they eat fish and shellfish that have lived in water with this kind of pollution. When fish and other creatures die from petroleum pollution, their bodies decay and release germs.

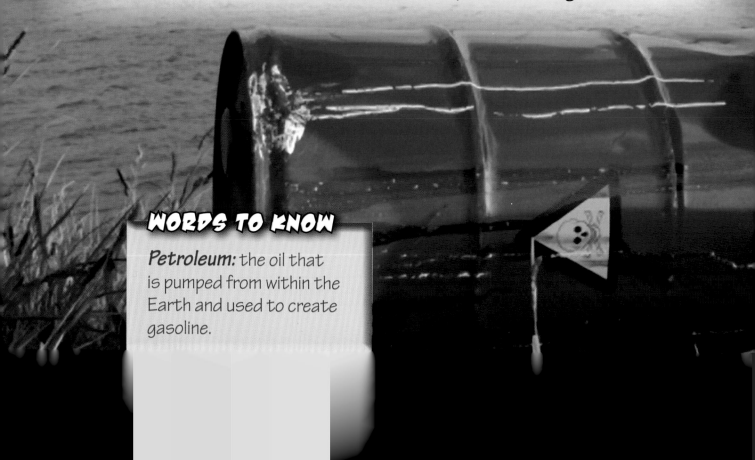

WORDS TO KNOW

Petroleum: the oil that is pumped from within the Earth and used to create gasoline.

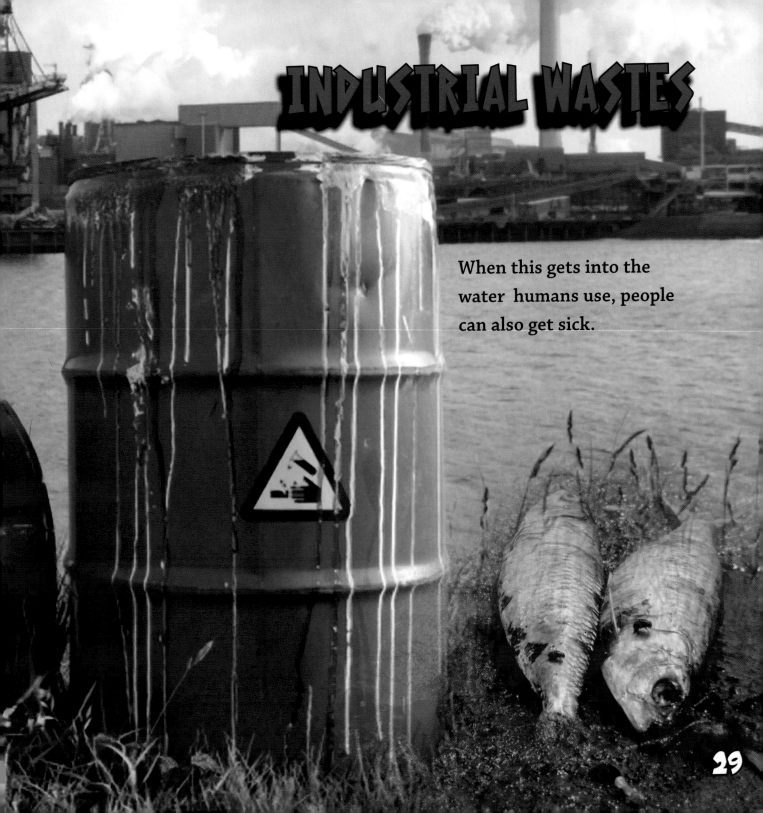

INDUSTRIAL WASTES

When this gets into the water humans use, people can also get sick.

RADIOACTIVE POLLUTION

Radioactive pollution comes from nuclear power plants and nuclear weapons. However, medical facilities and industries also release radioactive pollution into the Earth's waterways. These waste products are very dangerous to Nature—and to humans.

Things that are radioactive can damage the DNA in animals and humans, which can cause birth defects and other abnormal growths. They can also cause cancer.

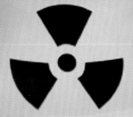

Radioactive waste is usually tasteless, odorless, and invisible. But it can be deadly to life on our planet. What's more it doesn't go away quickly—some kinds of radioactive waste can linger in the environmnet for as long as 600 years.

ASK THE DOCTOR

I've heard people say that nuclear power plants produce "clean" energy. Is that true?

A: Although nuclear power plants don't produce the kind of pollution that coal and oil does, waste from these plants can cause leukemia, thyroid cancer, bone cancer, and other forms of cancer. If an accident should happen at a nuclear power plant, the danger to human life would be immense. Because of this, nuclear power plants should not be considered a safe answer to our energy problems.

WORDS TO KNOW

Radioactive: giving off energy from atoms, which is something that some chemical elements do.

DNA: the material found within cells which passes along genes from parents to offspring.

Fetuses: developing humans inside their mothers before birth.

INSIDE

Radioactive waste can make cells grow in strange ways, causing cancerous tumors. It can get inside your bones and cause bone cancer. It can damage the growth of fetuses inside their mothers.

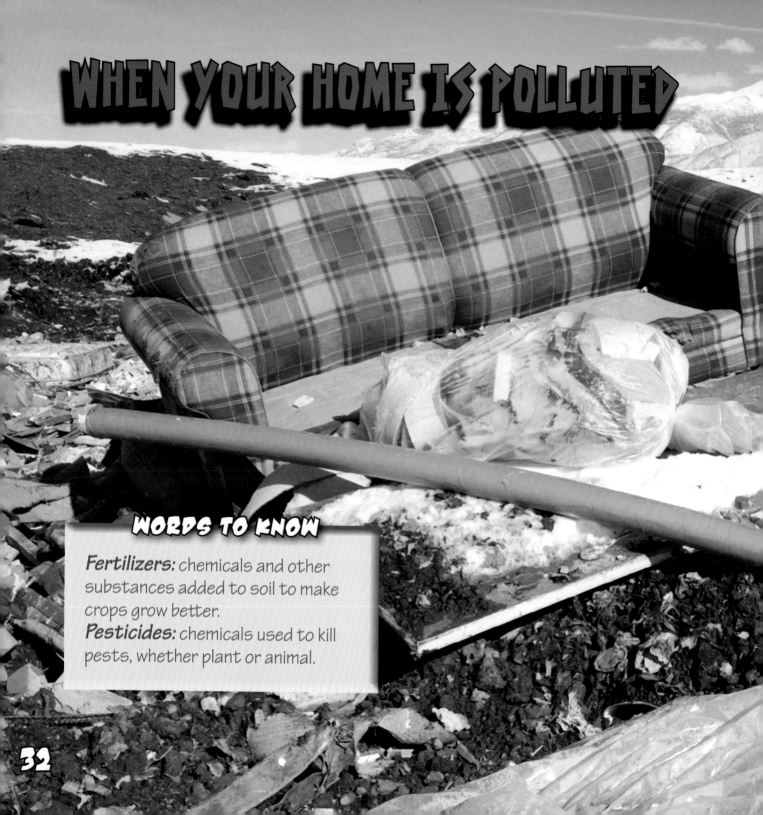

WHEN YOUR HOME IS POLLUTED

WORDS TO KNOW

Fertilizers: chemicals and other substances added to soil to make crops grow better.

Pesticides: chemicals used to kill pests, whether plant or animal.

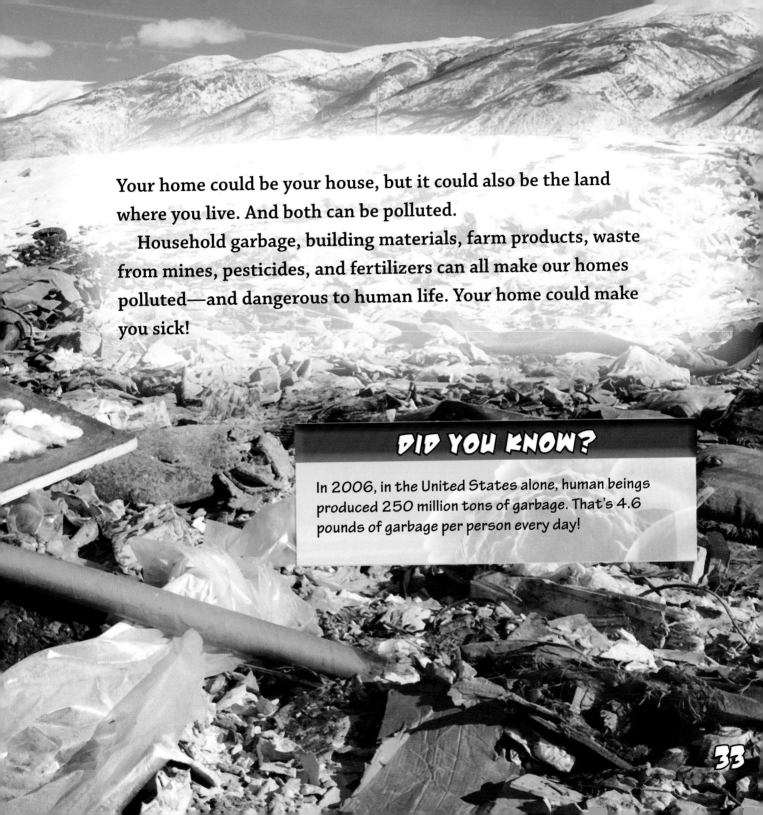

Your home could be your house, but it could also be the land where you live. And both can be polluted.

Household garbage, building materials, farm products, waste from mines, pesticides, and fertilizers can all make our homes polluted—and dangerous to human life. Your home could make you sick!

DID YOU KNOW?

In 2006, in the United States alone, human beings produced 250 million tons of garbage. That's 4.6 pounds of garbage per person every day!

POLLUTED HOUSES

DANGER
Do Not Enter
Asbestos Contaminated
Area
For Information Call City Property •

34

Pollution isn't something you find only in the outdoors. It can also be found indoors, inside a house. Mold is one kind of indoor pollution. When carpets and walls are moist, mold can grow on them. This mold releases spores into the air. When you breathe, you suck the spores inside your lungs, where they can give you breathing problems. They can also cause different kinds of allergies that may make you itchy, headachy, or grouchy. Another kind of indoor pollution comes from asbestos, a mineral that used to be used in insulation and other building materials. Nowadays, this material is no longer used, but it can still be found in older buildings. If you inhale asbestos fibers, it can cause lung cancer.

WORDS TO KNOW

Spores: the tiny particles from which new mold grows.

35

POLLUTED SOIL

The Earth's soil can become polluted from several different sources. Here are a few of the ways:

• Buried waste containers can break.

• Pesticides and fertilizers can get into the soil from farms.

• Water that runs through landfills and garbage dumps can carry pollution into soil.

• Factories dump chemicals and other waste products directly into the ground.

• Acid rain carries chemical pollution in the air to the earth.

WORDS TO KNOW

Landfills: places where trash and garbage are buried beneath layers of dirt.

Soil pollution can be dangerous to people, especially children who often play in parks and playgrounds where they touch dirt. Some chemicals found in soil pollution can cause cancers. Others, such as lead, can damage kidneys. Lead poisoning can also damage children's brains and keep them from developing normally.

DID YOU KNOW?

Lead poisoning can come from outside your outdoor home, from the soil—but it can also be found sometimes in your indoor home, especially if you live in an older home. Lead used to be used in paint and in water pipes. Young children who put things in their mouths are especially apt to get lead poisoning if they live in a house where old paint is chipping off the walls.

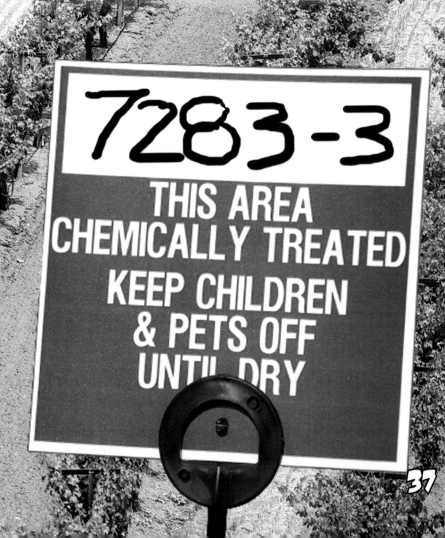

7283-3

THIS AREA
CHEMICALLY TREATED
KEEP CHILDREN
& PETS OFF
UNTIL DRY

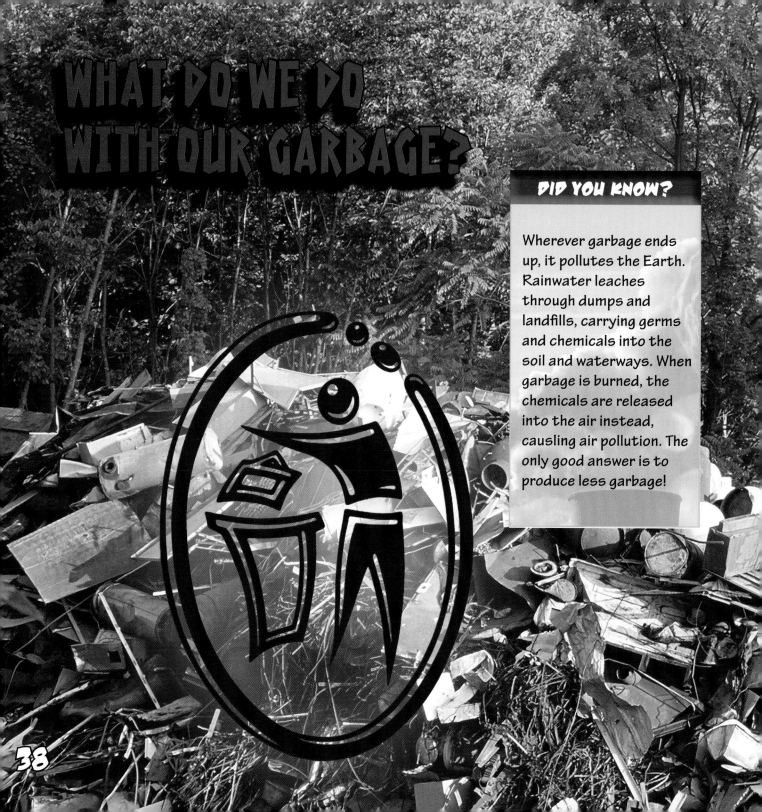

WHAT DO WE DO WITH OUR GARBAGE?

38

DID YOU KNOW?

Wherever garbage ends up, it pollutes the Earth. Rainwater leaches through dumps and landfills, carrying germs and chemicals into the soil and waterways. When garbage is burned, the chemicals are released into the air instead, causling air pollution. The only good answer is to produce less garbage!

Finding a place to put our garbage is a big problem. In the days before plastic, the problem wasn't as serious. Left to nature, leftover food, paper, and wood products eventually break down and go back into the soil. Plastic is a different thing altogether—it NEVER breaks down. Unless it's burned (which releases toxic chemicals into the air), that plastic candy wrapper you threw into the garbage today will still be around a hundred years from now. In fact, it will still be around a thousand years from now!

When you throw something in a waste basket, you probably never give it another thought. But think about all the millions of people in the world, all producing garbage of one sort or another every day. Where does all that garbage go?

Sometimes it goes to dumps, like the one shown in this picture. Sometimes it goes into landfills. Sometimes it goes into the oceans. Other times it gets burned in incinerators. Once in a while, it goes on a flat boat and floats around the world, looking for someplace willing to take it!

WORDS TO KNOW

Leaches: washes water or another liquid through a substance, dissolving some of the substance in the process.

GLOBAL WARMING AND YOUR BODY

ASK THE DOCTOR

My mom says that growing plants make us healthier. Is that true?

A: Your mother is right. Plants take in carbon dioxide and give off oxygen. That's the opposite from us: we breathe in oxygen and release carbon dioxide. So plants and animals are the perfect balance for each other on our planet. Destroying acres of forests contributes to global warming. But keeping plenty of plants in your house can actually improve the quality of your air.

OUTSIDE YOUR BODY

Global warming is caused by the buildup of "greenhouse gases"—mostly carbon dioxide—in the atmosphere. These gases form a sort of blanket over the Earth, trapping in heat that would normally escape the atmosphere. When coal, oil, and gas are burned in our factories, vehicles, and homes, they release carbon dioxide into the air. This change in the Earth's atmosphere is also changing the Earth's climates.

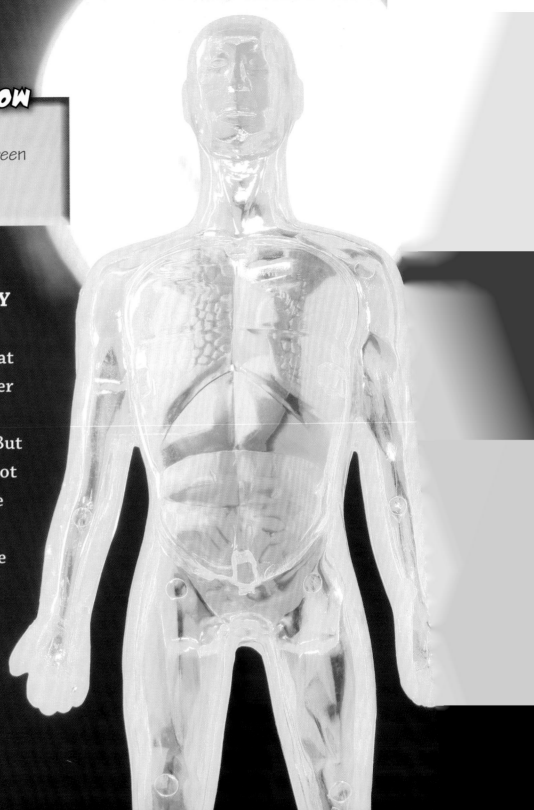

WORDS TO KNOW

Carbon dioxide: a colorless gas that green plants use to create food.

INSIDE YOUR BODY

You may not think that if the Earth gets hotter it will matter all that much to human life. But scientists say that's not the case. Our lives are tied so closely to the Earth that any change in our planet's health affects our health as well. Climate change can make us sick in four main ways.

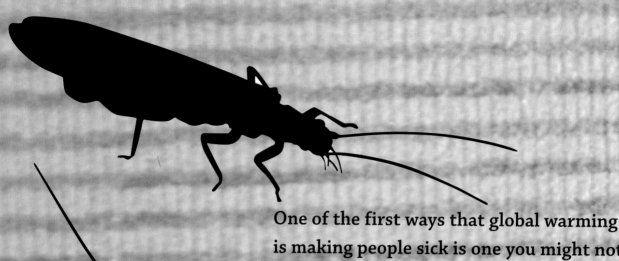

One of the first ways that global warming is making people sick is one you might not think of. But as temperatures get higher, certain kinds of insects reproduce more quickly. Frost and cold temperatures normally kill the larvae of flies, mosquitoes, and fleas. But as the climate changes, Nature's way to control insect populations will be destroyed. This means that there will be more mosquitoes, flies, and other insects in certain parts of the world.

ASK THE DOCTOR

My mother always says that flies are dirty and that they spread disease. Is that true?

A: Yes, it's true. Because flies crawl on and eat dead flesh and fecal material, they carry germs on their feet, which can then spread to whatever else they crawl on.

INSECTS THAT SPREAD DISEASE

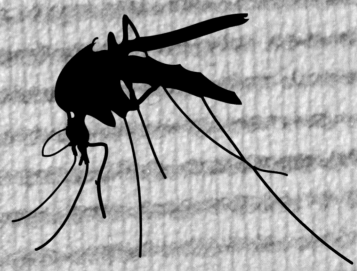

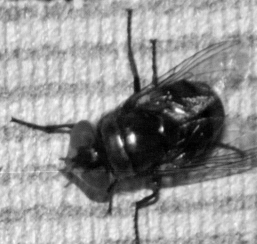

Especially in parts of Africa, Asia, and South America, mosquitoes carry malaria and other diseases. Tics in North America spread Lyme disease. Other insects can carry other sicknesses. As the Earth's temperature goes up, the numbers of these insects will increase as well—and more people will get sick.

WORDS TO KNOW

Larvae: one of the stages in the life of an insect; when an insect's egg "hatches" the little "worms" that come out are called larvae.

INCREASED AIR POLLUTION

ASK THE DOCTOR

I live in the country. Do I need to worry about air pollution?

A: Air quality is usually better in the country than in urban areas where there are lots of cars and factories. But think about sitting in the No Smoking section of a restaurant or other public place. If someone is smoking, even on the other side of the room, eventually that smoke spreads to the No Smoking section.

The same thing happens with the Earth's air. Pollution doesn't pay any attention to cities' or nations' borders; air pollution spreads through the atmosphere; it doesn't stay put but seeps around the planet. And global warming affects the entire planet's atmosphere, both rural areas and urban. Pollution is the entire Earth's problem.

The "greenhouse effect" that causes the Earth's temperature to rise also acts like a lid on a pot, holding in the air pollution so it can't escape. This means that ozone and other chemicals build up in the air we breathe. This can be dangerous to your health.

How dangerous it is depends on who you are and how much ozone is in the air. Most people only have to worry about ozone exposure when ground-level concentrations reach high levels. In many cities, this can happen frequently during the summer months. In general, as ground-level ozone concentrations increase, more and more people will feel sick, the effects become more serious, and more people are

WORDS TO KNOW

Concentration: how much there is of something in another substance. When concentration is high, there's a lot of whatever it is.

admitted to the hospital for respiratory problems. Ozone can irritate the lining of your lungs. It can make people who already have asthma feel worse. Ozone can also make it so you can't breathe in as much air, which means your body has less oxygen. This in turn will effect how your entire body feels and how well it can function. If you breathe air that has lots of ozone in it for long periods of time, it can permanently damage the lungs.

People who are very young, very old, or who have breathing problems already are most apt to get sick from breathing lots of ozone. When ozone levels are very high, everyone should worry about ozone exposure. This means people should avoid exercising outdoors. They should stay inside as much as possible.

Doctors say that ozone hurts the inside of the lungs in a way that's a lot like getting a bad sunburn on your skin. Ozone damages the cells that line the air spaces in the lung. Within a few days, the damaged cells are replaced and the old cells are shed, much in the way that skin peels after a sunburn. If this kind of damage occurs repeatedly, the lung may change permanently in a way that could cause long-term health effects and a lower quality of life.

DID YOU KNOW?

SMOKE + FOG = SMOG

The word "smog" was first used by Dr. Henry Antoine Des Voeux in 1905 in a paper he wrote called "Fog and Smoke," for a meeting of the Public Health Congress. The 26 July 1905 edition of the London newspaper *Daily Graphic* quoted Des Voeux, "He said it required no science to see that there was something produced in great cities which was not found in the country, and that was smoky fog, or what was known as 'smog.'" The following day the newspaper stated that "Dr. Des Voeux did a public service in coining a new word for the London fog."

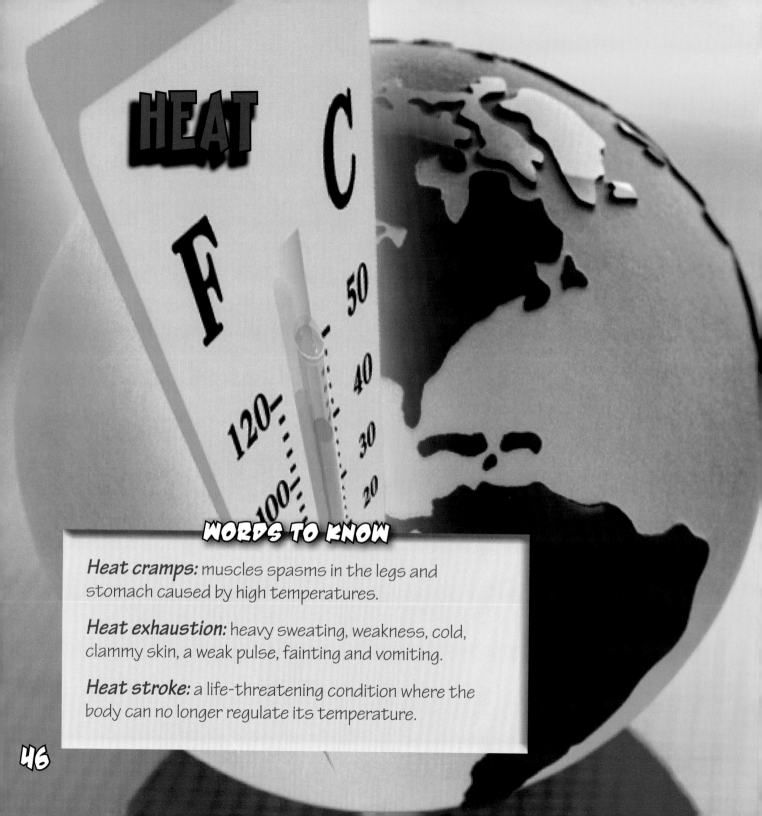

HEAT

WORDS TO KNOW

Heat cramps: muscles spasms in the legs and stomach caused by high temperatures.

Heat exhaustion: heavy sweating, weakness, cold, clammy skin, a weak pulse, fainting and vomiting.

Heat stroke: a life-threatening condition where the body can no longer regulate its temperature.

46

Global warming not only causes the Earth's average temperature to go up by a few degrees—it also is causing heat waves to be more frequent around the globe.

A heat wave is an extended interval of abnormally hot and unusually humid weather. It usually lasts from a few days to over a week.

Heat waves are dangerous to our health. Heat makes the human body have to work harder than it does normally. This causes stress and weakness. Eventually, it can even cause death.

Older people whose hearts are already tired or sick are most likely to suffer serious health consequences during heat waves. When these people do not have air conditioning or anywhere they can go to escape the heat, they are most in danger.

On very hot days, try to give your body a break. Don't exercise as much or as hard. Find some place cooler, even if it's only the shade from a tree. Go swimming if you can. Give yourself permission to be lazy. Your body will thank you!

DID YOU KNOW?

When the temperature is 130 degrees or higher: heatstroke/sunstroke is highly likely.

When the temperature is 105–130 degrees: sunstroke, heat cramps, or heat exhaustion are likely if you stay in the heat for very long.

When the temperature is 90–105 degrees: sunstroke, heat cramps, and heat exhaustion are possible if you stay outside long or exercise in the heat.

When the temperature is 80–90 degrees: you may feel very tired if you stay in the heat for very long or exercise in the heat.

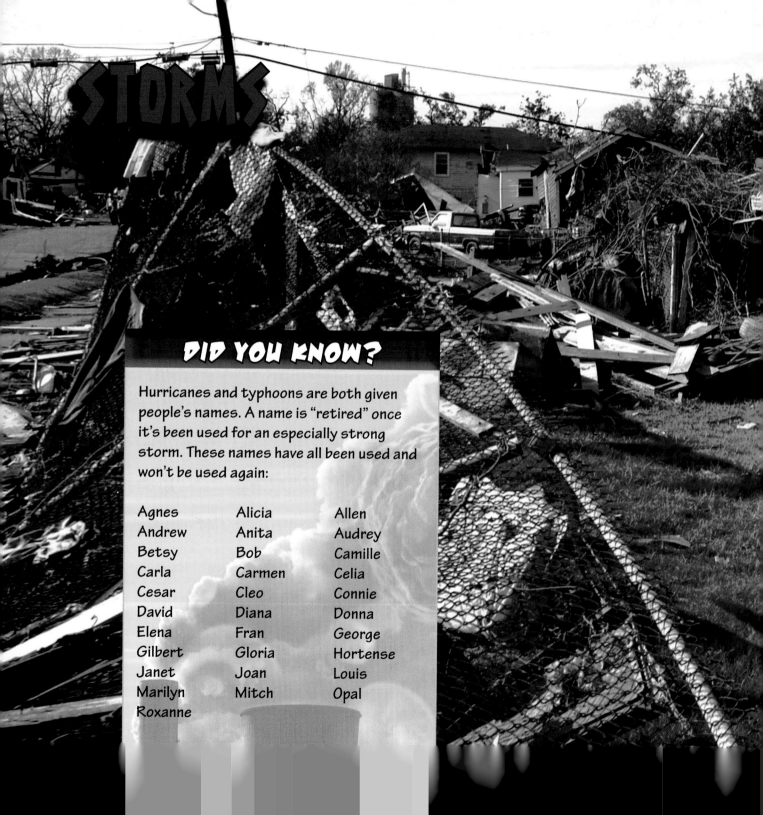

STORMS

DID YOU KNOW?

Hurricanes and typhoons are both given people's names. A name is "retired" once it's been used for an especially strong storm. These names have all been used and won't be used again:

Agnes	Alicia	Allen
Andrew	Anita	Audrey
Betsy	Bob	Camille
Carla	Carmen	Celia
Cesar	Cleo	Connie
David	Diana	Donna
Elena	Fran	George
Gilbert	Gloria	Hortense
Janet	Joan	Louis
Marilyn	Mitch	Opal
Roxanne		

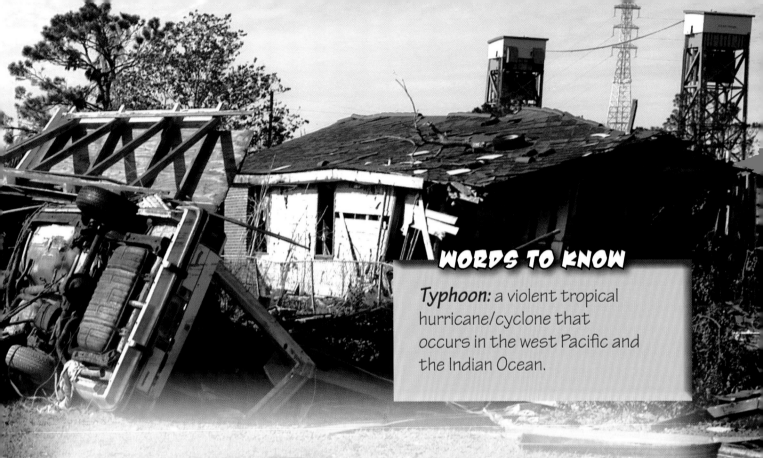

WORDS TO KNOW

Typhoon: a violent tropical hurricane/cyclone that occurs in the west Pacific and the Indian Ocean.

In the last few years, people have noticed that there have been more severe hurricanes and typhoons than ever before. Scientists suspect that global warming is to blame.

Global warming doesn't create hurricanes, but it does make them stronger and more dangerous. Because the ocean is getting warmer, tropical storms can pick up more energy and become more powerful. So global warming could turn a smaller storm into a bigger storm. Researchers have found that hurricanes and typhoons have become more dangerous and destructive as ocean temperatures have risen over the past 35 years.

DROUGHT

A drought is an extended period of months or years when a region doesn't have enough water. Usually this happens when there's not enough rain or other precipitation. When this happens, it can have very bad effects on the balance of the ecosystem.

In some regions of the world, droughts have lasted for years and years. When this happens, wildlife dies and farms grow no food. Sometimes people starve. This is what's been happening in parts of Africa during the past decades.

Some droughts only last a few weeks—but even those can damage farmland and wildlife.

Scientists say that every year an area of fertile soil the size of the nation of Ukraine (or the U.S. state of Texas) is lost because of drought.

Drought is a normal climate pattern in some parts of the world—but global warming is making droughts come more often and last longer. In many parts of Africa, people are suffering and sometimes dying. Food and water shortages also trigger conflcts and violence.

WORDS TO KNOW

Decade: ten-year period.

The problem could get even worse. Scientists say that as mountain glaciers melt in the Earth's rising temperatures, some of the world's biggest rivers (which are fed by the mountain glaciers) could also disappear. Without these water sources, people will have nowhere to go for water for irrigation and household use during times of little rainfall. The rainforest could die. Without the Earth's millions of trees, our atmosphere will suffer even more.

Global warming is a serious problem. We can't ignore it and hope it goes away. We have to do something! And we have to do it now!

DID YOU KNOW?

Drought has many short-term and long-term effects for both humans and Nature. It can cause:

- forest fires
- malnutrition
- unemployment
- destruction of wildlife species
- increased poverty
- population migrations (movements) to different places

WHAT SHOULD WE DO?

By reducing pollution from vehicles and power plants. Right away, we should put existing technologies for building cleaner cars and more modern electricity generators into widespread use. We can increase our reliance on renewable energy sources such as wind, sun and geothermal. And we can manufacture more efficient appliances and conserve energy

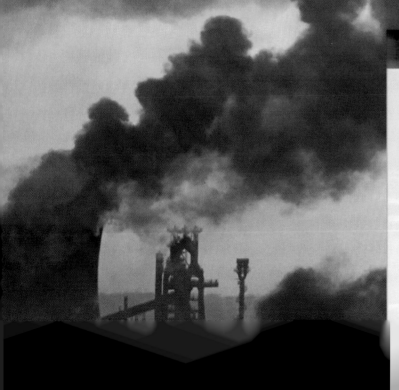

DID YOU KNOW?

If we all changed the way we lived in simple ways, we could help save the environment. For instance, using wind energy is better for the air than burning coal to make electricity. if you eat food that is grown locally, instead of being shipped from across the world, you cut down on the greenhouse gases that would have been put in the atmosphere transporting the food. So even the way you eat can make a big difference to our planet!

A Story From Real Life

Africa's Lake Tanganyika, the longest fresh water lake in the world and the second deepest, provides homes and food for a variety of living creatures, including human beings, who rely on the lake's fish for sustenance. Many of Tanganyika's 350 species of fish live nowhere else on Earth, because the lake offers a unique ecosystem: up until recently, its temperature has been almost uniformly consistent, even in its deepest water, 4,700 feet down. Unfortunately, global warming may be affecting Lake Tanganyika. Even a few degrees difference in temperature kills fish—and affects the livelihoods of millions of people.

Seph, a fisherman on Lake Tanganyika, said that fishing is much more difficult now than it was thirty years ago when he was a teenager. "Oh, it was so good," he said. "When we used to fish with our fathers, it was really good. There were so many dagaa [a type of sardine]. People could fish five thousand tons. In tons! Back in those days there was so much dagaa."

The people who live on Lake Tanganyika's shore rely on Nature for their livelihoods. Seph said, "We fish because we have no other job. Our grandfathers fished here. Our fathers fished here. We'll fish here and pass it on to our children who will fish and pass it on again. It's our legacy."

If the fish disappear, what legacy will Seph—and the fishers of other waters around the world—leave to their children?

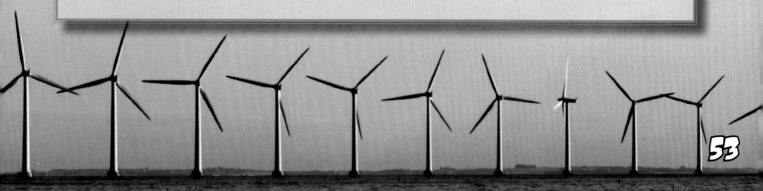

WHAT IS THE WORLD DOING?

On 11 December 1997, many of the world's nations met in Kyoto, Japan, to talk about what could be done to reduce greenhouse gases that cause climate change. As of November 2007, 175 parties have ratified the protocol. Of these, 36 developed countries (plus all the countries in the European Union) and 139 developing countries have promised to reduce greenhouse gas emissions. The world knows this is a big problem. Scientists, governments, and ordinary people are all getting involved.

Protecting the Earth means we all need to change the way we live. We can no longer use things and throw them away. We can no longer burn gas and oil and coal to run our cars and factories. We have to find new ways of doing things!

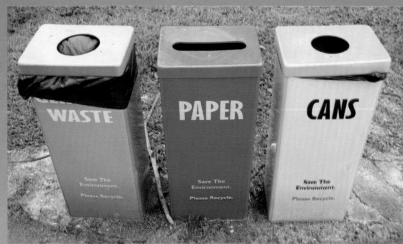

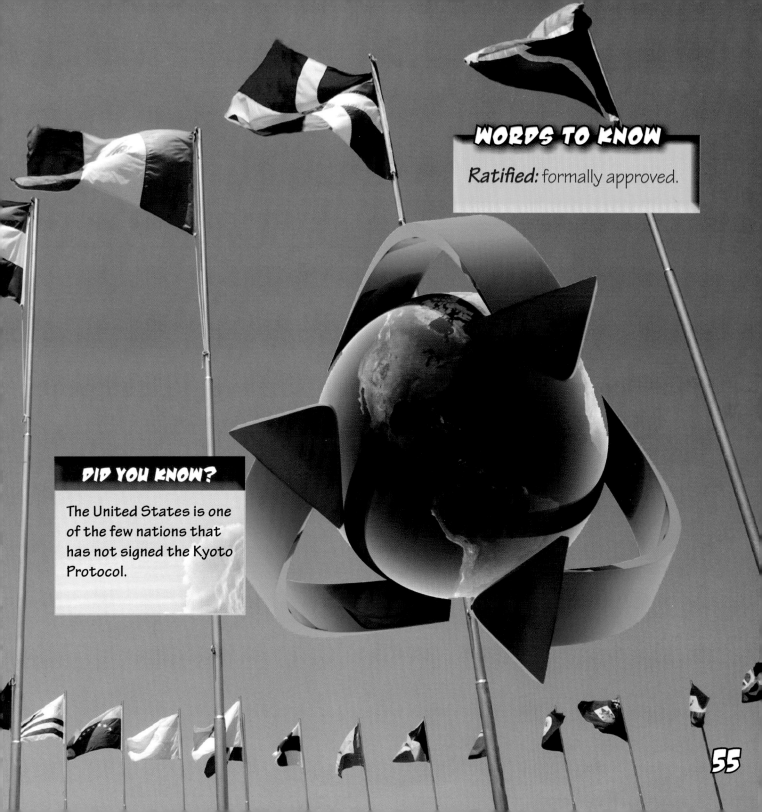

WORDS TO KNOW

Ratified: formally approved.

DID YOU KNOW?

The United States is one of the few nations that has not signed the Kyoto Protocol.

WHAT CAN YOU DO?

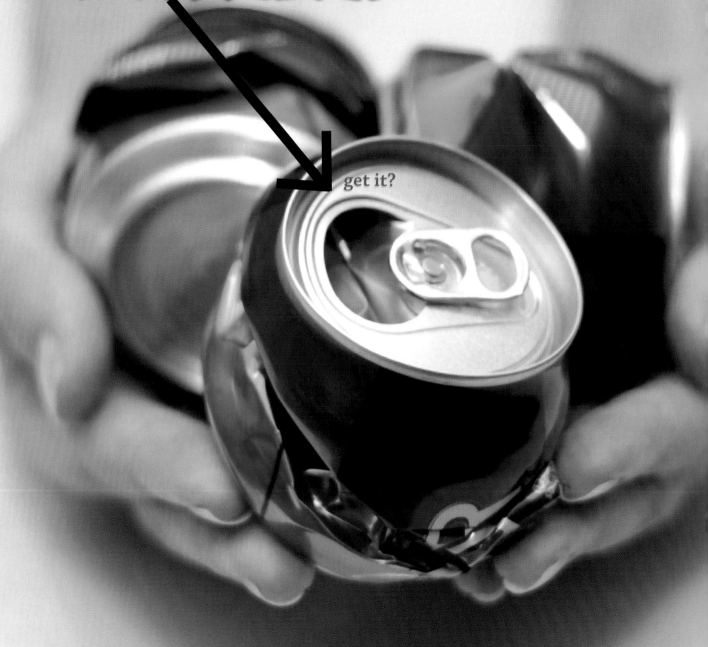

get it?

Waste is anything thrown away into the environment in a manner (or quantity) that could have an impact on that environment. How can you help? By practicing the three R's of waste management: **REDUCE, REUSE, RECYCLE!**

REDUCE

Buy and use less! Start making wise "package" selections. Refuse store bags. Use durable items rather than disposable items whenever possible.

REUSE

Use cloth gift bags instead of wrapping paper or paper gift bags. Use cloth napkins instead of paper napkins. Share outgrown clothes with people who need them—or have a yard sale.

RECYCLE

Don't throw things away—take them to a recycling center instead. Just about anything in your home (or office or school, etc.) that cannot be reused CAN be recycled into something else. You'd be amazed what can be done with a recycled product. A recycled soda bottle, for example, can be made into T-shirts, combs, or hundreds of other plastic goods that can be used for many years.

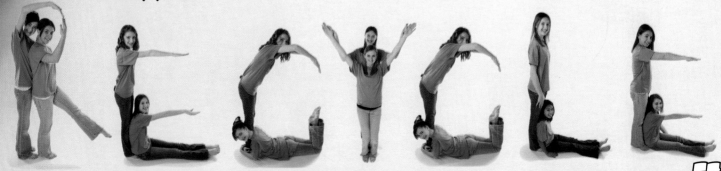

If we want to save our planet—and keep ourselves healthy as well—we all have to do our part. The Earth's health can't be separated from our own! We must all do what we can to protect our air and water and land. Here are some things you can do:

Walk or ride your bicycle instead of getting a ride. Plant trees that put oxygen back into the air. Use more efficient light bulbs. Turn off lights when you're not using them. Unplug appliances not in use. Be an ecologist.

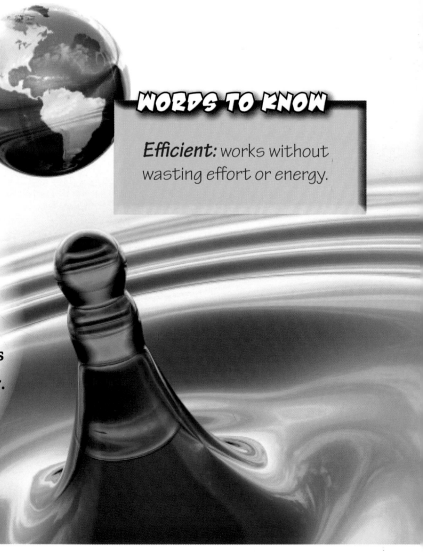

WORDS TO KNOW

Efficient: works without wasting effort or energy.

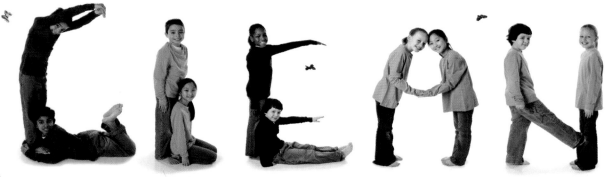

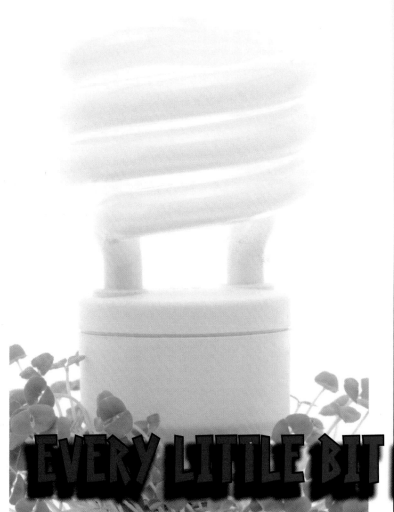

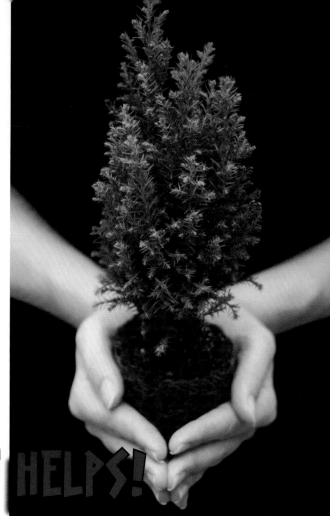

EVERY LITTLE BIT HELPS!

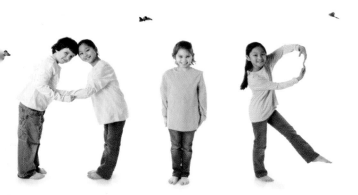

WORDS TO KNOW

Ecologist: a person who studies the relationship of living things to each other and to what's around them.

Consumer Healthcare Products Association
www.chpa-info.org/ChpaPortal/PressRoom/FAQs/Dextromethorphan.htm

Focus Adolescent Services
www.focusas.com/SubstanceAbuse.html

Go Ask Alice
www.goaskalice.columbia.edu

Health Canada
www.hc-sc.gc.ca/index_e.html

Parents. The Anti-Drug.
www.theantidrug.com

The Partnership for a Drug-Free America
www.drugfree.org/Parent
Parents: www.drugfree.org/dxm
Teens: www.dxmstories.com

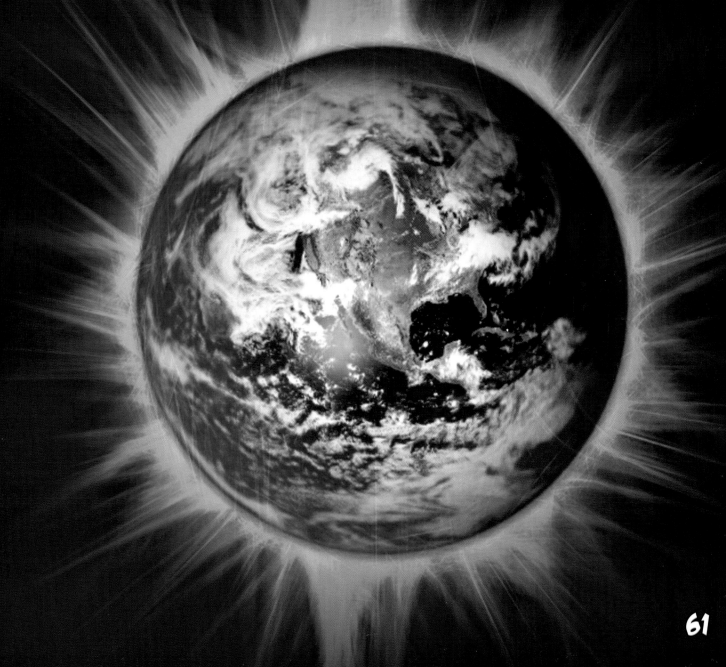

Rader Programs—Specializing in the Treatment of Anorexia, Bulimia, and Compulsive Overeating

www.raderprograms.com/index.aspx

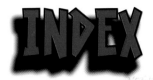

INDEX

Africa 16, 25, 43, 50, 53
air pollution 8, 9, 12, 14-17, 19, 20, 38, 44
Asia 25, 43
asthma 15-17, 45
atmosphere 40, 44, 51, 52

cancer 15, 20, 21, 30, 31, 35, 37
chemical 8, 9, 12, 16, 20, 22, 26, 31, 32, 36-39, 44
climate 40, 41, 42, 50, 54
coal 15, 31, 40, 52, 54

disease 15, 17-20, 25, 42, 43

Earth 8, 9, 11, 13, 27, 28, 30, 36, 38, 40-44, 47, 51, 53, 54, 58
energy 31, 49, 52, 58
excercise 14, 17, 19, 47

fish 22, 26-28, 53

garbage 9, 11, 26, 33, 36, 38, 39
germ 23, 25, 28, 38, 42
global warming 8, 13, 40, 42, 47, 49-51, 53

heart 15, 18, 19, 47
hurricane 48, 49

land pollution 8, 12
lead 16, 19, 21, 23, 37

leukemia 20, 31
lung 11, 14-18, 20, 21, 35, 45
lyme disease 43

insect 22, 42, 43

malaria 43
mercury 26,27

nature 8, 22, 30, 39, 42, 51, 53

ocean 26, 28, 39, 49
oil 8, 28, 31, 36-40, 50, 54
ozone 16, 17, 44, 45

pneumonia 15

radioactive 30

South America 43
stroke 15, 46, 47

toxic 20, 21, 39
typhoon 48, 49

water pollution 8, 13, 22
wildlife 8, 22, 28 50, 51
wood 15, 39

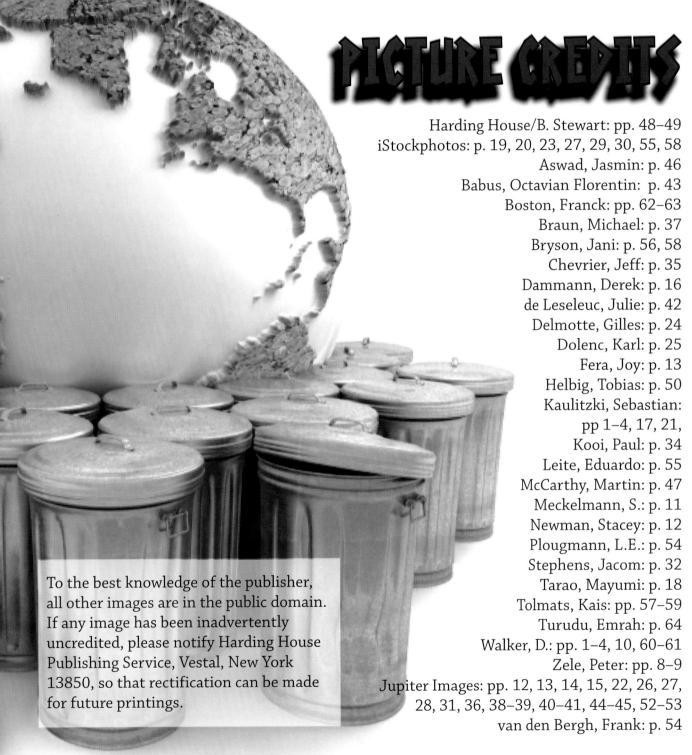

PICTURE CREDITS

Harding House/B. Stewart: pp. 48–49
iStockphotos: p. 19, 20, 23, 27, 29, 30, 55, 58
Aswad, Jasmin: p. 46
Babus, Octavian Florentin: p. 43
Boston, Franck: pp. 62–63
Braun, Michael: p. 37
Bryson, Jani: p. 56, 58
Chevrier, Jeff: p. 35
Dammann, Derek: p. 16
de Leseleuc, Julie: p. 42
Delmotte, Gilles: p. 24
Dolenc, Karl: p. 25
Fera, Joy: p. 13
Helbig, Tobias: p. 50
Kaulitzki, Sebastian:
pp 1–4, 17, 21,
Kooi, Paul: p. 34
Leite, Eduardo: p. 55
McCarthy, Martin: p. 47
Meckelmann, S.: p. 11
Newman, Stacey: p. 12
Plougmann, L.E.: p. 54
Stephens, Jacom: p. 32
Tarao, Mayumi: p. 18
Tolmats, Kais: pp. 57–59
Turudu, Emrah: p. 64
Walker, D.: pp. 1–4, 10, 60–61
Zele, Peter: pp. 8–9
Jupiter Images: pp. 12, 13, 14, 15, 22, 26, 27,
28, 31, 36, 38–39, 40–41, 44–45, 52–53
van den Bergh, Frank: p. 54

To the best knowledge of the publisher, all other images are in the public domain. If any image has been inadvertently uncredited, please notify Harding House Publishing Service, Vestal, New York 13850, so that rectification can be made for future printings.

ABOUT THE AUTHOR

Rae Simons has written many books for young adults and children. After writing this book, she has become convinced that she and her family need to do more to help protect the environment.

ABOUT THE CONSULTANT

Elise DeVore Berlan, MD, MPH, FAAP, is a faculty member of the Division of Adolescent Health at Nationwide Children's Hospital and an Assistant Professor of Clinical Pediatrics at The Ohio State University College of Medicine. She completed her Fellowship in Adolescent Medicine at Children's Hospital Boston and obtained a Master's Degree in Public Health at the Harvard School of Public Health. Dr. Berlan completed her residency in pediatrics at the Children's Hospital of Philadelphia, where she also served an additional year as Chief Resident. She received her medical degree from the University of Iowa College of Medicine. Dr. Berlan is board certified in Pediatrics and board eligible in Adolescent Medicine. She provides primary care and consultative services in the area of Young Women's Health, including gynecological problems, concerns about puberty, reproductive health services, and reproductive endocrine disorders.